Table of Contents

Pulmonary Fibrosis (PF) is a type of rare lung disease that causes the tissue (interstitium) around the air sacs (alveoli) within the lungs to become thickened and scarred – this is called fibrosis. This scarring makes the lungs stiff which makes it increasingly difficult to breathe deeply. This stops the efficient delivery of oxygen into the bloodstream where it is needed to be transported to the rest of the body.

There are many types of PF. Some people with PF may already have features of other associated conditions such as rheumatoid arthritis or scleroderma. Idiopathic Pulmonary Fibrosis (IPF) is a specific disease where the underlying cause is unknown. It is important for your healthcare team to identify the underlying type of PF, to help determine the most appropriate treatment options for your condition. These webpages provide information that is common across the different types of PF. For information that is specific to your diagnosis, it is important that you speak with your healthcare team.

Pulmonary fibrosis is a progressive disease that causes lung tissue to become thickened and scarred. This scarring makes the lungs stiff, making it increasingly difficult to breathe deeply. It can be easy to dismiss the common symptoms of pulmonary fibrosis as ageing or lack of fitness but breathlessness, cough, fatigue and unexplained weight loss shouldn't be ignored. Early diagnosis and treatment can help slow disease progression and improve quality of life. Learn more about pulmonary fibrosis and talk to your GP today.

Researchers currently believe that a combination of exposure to lung irritants like certain chemicals, smoking, and infections, along with genetics and immune system activity, play key roles in pulmonary fibrosis.

It was once thought that the condition was caused by inflammation. Now scientists believe that there is an abnormal healing process in the lungs that leads to scarring. The formation of significant lung scarring eventually becomes pulmonary fibrosis.

BREAKFAST

1. Crustless Quiche

Prep Time: 20 Minutes

Cook Time: 40 Minutes

Servings: 4

Ingredients

- 2 cups shredded cheddar cheese
- 5-ounce can evaporated milk or 2/3 cup heavy whipping cream
- 1 cup small broccoli florets
- 4 strips bacon
- 3 large eggs
- 3 scallions, sliced (1/3 cup)
- 1 tomato, sliced
- 1 teaspoon dried basil
- 1/4 teaspoon ground black pepper

Instructions

1. Prepare: Preheat oven to 350 F. Grease and set aside 9-inch pie dish.

2. Pre-Cook Ingredients: Microwave broccoli until tender, a few minutes, and drain on paper towels. Microwave bacon strips according to package instructions until crispy, about 5 minutes, or pan fry them. When cool, crumble bacon into small pieces.

3. Assemble Quiche: Evenly distribute ingredients over pie dish in this order: 1/3 of shredded cheese, broccoli, 1/3 of shredded cheese, bacon, scallions, then remaining 1/3 of shredded cheese. Beat together milk (or cream), eggs, basil, and black pepper in bowl until combined, then pour over ingredients in pie dish. Decorate top of quiche with sliced tomatoes.

4. Bake & Cool: Bake quiche at 350 F for 40 minutes. Cool for 15 minutes before cutting into 4 slices, then serve.

Prep Time: 30 Minutes

Cook Time: 60 Minutes

Servings: 6

Ingredients

Meat Layer:

- 1 pound ground lamb
- 1 cup diced celery
- 1/2 cup diced onions
- 1/2 cup diced carrots
- 1 cup beef broth
- 3 tablespoons tomato paste
- 1 tablespoon olive oil
- 1.5 teaspoons dried rosemary leaves
- 1.5 teaspoons table salt
- 1 teaspoon ground thyme
- 1/2 teaspoon ground black pepper

Mashed Cauliflower Layer:

- 1.5 pounds cauliflower florets
- 1/2 cup shredded cheddar cheese

- 2 ounces cream cheese, softened to room temperature
- 2 tablespoons salted butter, softened to room temperature
- 2 cloves garlic, minced
- 1/4 teaspoon table salt
- 1/4 teaspoon ground black pepper

Optional Toppings:

- Shredded cheddar cheese
- Smoked paprika
- Olive oil
- Chives or parsley

Instructions

1. Sauté: Heat olive oil in large pan over medium-high heat. Add meat and cook until no longer pink, about 5 minutes, crumbling with wooden spoon. Add diced celery, onions, carrots, rosemary, thyme, salt, and pepper to pan. Cook until vegetables soften, about 5 minutes, stirring occasionally.

2. Simmer Meat Sauce: Add beef broth and tomato paste to same pan, stirring until paste dissolves. Reduce heat slightly and continue simmering until sauce thickens,

about 15 minutes. While simmering, start preparing mashed cauliflower in next step.

3. Cook Cauliflower: Microwave cauliflower florets in large microwave-safe bowl until very tender, about 10 minutes. Spread out florets on paper towels to drain for 5 to 10 minutes, or until steaming subsides.

4. Purée Cauliflower: Transfer cauliflower to food processor. Add cheddar cheese, cream cheese, butter, garlic, salt, and pepper. Purée until mixture has smooth consistency resembling mashed potatoes, pausing as needed to scrape down sides of food processor bowl.

5. Assemble Casserole: Use slotted spoon (so that any grease is left behind) to transfer meat sauce to 8×8 inch baking dish (Note 4), evenly spreading along bottom of dish. Evenly spread mashed cauliflower over meat sauce. Use fork to roughen cauliflower surface. Optionally, top with shredded cheddar cheese and paprika, and lightly drizzle olive oil on top.

6. Bake: Bake at 400 F until peaks of mashed cauliflower are browning, about 30 minutes. Optionally, garnish with chives or parsley. Casserole will be very hot; cool in baking dish, then slice and serve.

Prep Time: 10 Minutes

Cook Time: 25 Minutes

Servings: 2

Ingredients

- 2.5 cups cauliflower rice
- 2/3 cup shredded cheddar cheese
- 1/4 cup almond flour
- 2 large eggs, unbeaten
- 1 scallion, thinly sliced
- 2 tablespoons butter
- 1/2 teaspoon table salt
- 1/4 teaspoon ground black pepper

Instructions

1. Cook Cauliflower Rice: Cover and microwave cauliflower rice until fully cooked and softened, about 4 minutes for fresh cauliflower, or 5 minutes for frozen cauliflower. Let cool for 5 minutes or until steaming subsides.

2. Make Cauliflower Mixture: Stir cooked cauliflower rice, cheddar cheese, almond flour, eggs, salt, and pepper in medium mixing bowl until well-mixed. Optionally, transfer mixture to colander set over bowl to allow excess liquid to drain while pan heats.

3. Cook Fritters: Spread butter on large pan over medium heat until melted, a few minutes. Use 1/4-cup measuring cup to scoop cauliflower mixture and overturn onto hot pan, immediately using spatula to flatten into 3 to 4 inch patty. Repeat until pan cannot hold any more in single layer, about 4 fritters. Cook each fritter until bottom is crispy and golden brown, about 5 minutes, then carefully flip with spatula to cook other side, another few minutes. Transfer to paper towel lined plate to drain. Repeat with second batch or until mixture is used up.

4. Cool & Serve: After cauliflower fritters have cooled on paper towels for about 10 minutes, transfer to serving plates and top with sliced scallions. Serve or save for later

Prep Time: 10 Minutes

Cook Time: 20 Minutes

Servings: 2

Ingredients

- 2/3 cup almond flour
- 3 tablespoons heavy whipping cream
- 3 tablespoons confectioners swerve sweetener
- 2 large egg whites
- 1/8 teaspoon table salt
- Butter and sugar-free syrup, for serving

Instructions

1. Make Batter: Stir together dry ingredients (almond flour, sweetener, salt) in a bowl until well-mixed. Stir in heavy cream and egg whites until batter is smooth. If batter is too thick, stir in 1 tablespoon of water.

2. Cook Pancakes: Heat a nonstick pan on the stove over medium-low until hot. Pour batter to form a 3-inch pancake, about 1 to 2 tablespoons. Cook until surface

bubbles are bursting, 1 to 2 minutes, and then flip to cook the other side until cooked through, another 30 seconds. Transfer to a plate when done. Repeat until batter is used up.

3. Serve: Serve immediately while hot, with butter and sugar-free syrup.

Prep Time: 15 Minutes

Cook Time: 15 Minutes

Servings: 4

Ingredients

- 8 large hard-boiled eggs, chopped
- 2 ripe avocados, chopped
- 2/3 cup diced celery (about 3 stalks)
- 2/3 cup sliced scallions (about 5 scallions)

Spicy Mayo Dressing:

- 1/2 cup mayonnaise
- 2 teaspoons dijon mustard
- 2 teaspoons smoked paprika
- 1/2 teaspoon ground cayenne
- 1/2 teaspoon ground black pepper
- 1/2 teaspoon table salt

Instructions

1. Make Dressing: Stir together all dressing ingredients in measuring glass or small bowl until very smooth.
2. Toss Salad: Toss chopped eggs, avocados, celery, scallions, and dressing in large salad bowl until well-mixed. Season with salt and pepper to taste. Cover and refrigerate until chilled. Serve or save for later.

6. Blueberry Scones

Prep Time: 15 Minutes

Cook Time: 20 Minutes

Servings: 6

Ingredients

- 1 cup blanched almond flour (4 ounces weight)
- 1/3 cup heavy whipping cream
- 2 tablespoons swerve sweetener (1 ounce weight)
- 1/4 cup fresh blueberries (1 ounce weight)
- 2 tablespoons coconut flour (1/2 ounce weight)
- 1/2 teaspoon baking powder
- 1/4 teaspoon salt

Instructions

1. Position a rack in the center of the oven. Preheat to 350 F. Prepare a baking tray lined with parchment paper or nonstick baking mat.
2. In a bowl, add dry ingredients (almond flour, sweetener, coconut flour, and baking powder, salt). Whisk until well-mixed.

3. Add heavy cream to the bowl. Stir together until absorbed and the mixture forms into a cohesive dough.
4. Add blueberries to the dough, carefully folding them in until well-distributed.
5. Divide the dough into 6 equal pieces. Form into wedge or triangle shapes. Space them out by 2-3 inches on the lined baking tray.
6. Bake at 350 F until the scones are lightly golden, 15 to 20 minutes.

Prep Time: 10 Minutes

Cook Time: 35 Minutes

Servings: 4

Ingredients

- 8 large eggs
- 6-ounce package baby spinach, roughly chopped
- 2 ounces prosciutto (4 slices), cut into 1 to 2 inch pieces
- 1 orange bell pepper, sliced into short strips
- 3/4 cup finely grated parmesan cheese, divided
- 1/2 cup heavy whipping cream
- 1 tablespoon olive oil
- 1/4 teaspoon ground black pepper
- 1/4 teaspoon table salt

Instructions

1. Make Egg Mixture: Whisk eggs, heavy cream, black pepper, salt, and half of parmesan cheese in large mixing bowl until well-beaten. Set aside.

2. Cook Prosciutto: Coat bottom of oven-safe 10-inch high-sided pan with olive oil, and add chopped prosciutto. Cook over medium heat until slightly crispy, 5 to 10 minutes, stirring occasionally. Use tongs to transfer prosciutto to large bowl, leaving behind oil and grease in pan.

3. Cook Vegetables: Add bell pepper slices to pan and cook until seared and soft, about 5 minutes, stirring occasionally. Transfer to same bowl with prosciutto. Reduce to medium-low heat. Add spinach to pan and cook until just wilted, a few minutes, stirring almost constantly. Transfer to same bowl. Turn off heat.

4. Assemble Frittata: Give egg mixture a stir and pour into pan. Leaving behind any juices in bowl, transfer prosciutto, spinach, and bell pepper to pan, arranging until evenly distributed in egg mixture. Gently push down on anything protruding up.

5. Cook Frittata: Cover with lid and cook over low heat until most of surface is no longer liquid, about 15 minutes. Gently shake pan; center should be set and only edges should be liquid. Remove pan from heat.

6. Broil Frittata: Uncover and evenly distribute remaining parmesan cheese on top. Optionally season with additional black pepper. Turn on broiler. Place

frittata in middle of oven and broil uncovered until surface is completely set and cheese is bubbling, 5 to 10 minutes. Frequently monitor so that frittata does not overcook.

7. Cool & Serve: Let stand to cool for a few minutes. Use spatula to loosen sides of frittata, then cut into wedges. Serve and save leftovers.

Prep Time: 10 Minutes

Cook Time: 15 Minutes

Servings: 4

Ingredients

- 4 low carb tortillas, brands like Mission or La Tortilla Factory
- 4 large eggs
- 1 large avocado
- 1/2 cup salsa
- 1/4 cup crumbled cheese, like cotija or feta
- 1 tablespoon olive oil
- Ground black pepper, to taste

Instructions

1. Warm Tortillas: Set aside sheet pan or 4 serving plates to hold tortillas. Heat skillet over medium heat until hot, a few minutes. One at a time, place tortilla on skillet and cook until warmed, about 1 minute per side, then transfer to prepared sheet pan or serving plates.

2. Cook Eggs: Add 1/2 tablespoon olive oil to now-empty skillet over medium heat. Crack 2 eggs on opposite sides of skillet, cooking until whites are nearly cooked through, 2 to 3 minutes. Flip eggs with spatula and cook another 30 seconds to firm up other side, then transfer to tortillas. Add remaining olive oil to pan, and repeat with remaining 2 eggs.

3. Add Toppings: Chop avocado and divide among tortillas. Spoon about 2 tablespoons of salsa and 1 tablespoon crumbled cheese onto each tortilla. Season with black pepper, and serve

Prep Time: 15 Minutes

Cook Time: 25 Minutes

Servings: 8

Ingredients

- 2 cups almond flour
- 1.5 cups shredded cheddar cheese
- 5 slices bacon, cooked and crumbled
- 2 large eggs
- 1/2 cup heavy whipping cream
- 2 tablespoons butter, diced
- 1 teaspoon table salt

Instructions

1. Prepare: Position oven rack in lower half of oven, and preheat to 375 F. Set aside baking half sheet lined with parchment paper or baking mat.
2. Make Dough: Stir almond flour and salt in large mixing bowl until well-mixed. Add cheese, eggs, cream, and

butter to bowl, stirring for a minute until well-mixed. Stir in crumbled bacon.

3. Bake: Evenly divide dough into 8 mounds on lined baking sheet, spaced 1 to 2 inches apart. Bake at 375 F until biscuits are browned and crispy, 25 to 30 minutes. Cool for 10 minutes and serve.

Prep Time: 5 Minutes

Cook Time: 30 Minutes

Servings: 5

Ingredients

- 2 large Russet potatoes about 2 pounds, peeled
- 4 slices bacon diced
- 3 scallions thinly sliced
- 1/2 teaspoon salt
- 1/2 teaspoon pepper
- 1/2 cup butter melted

Instructions

1. Run the potatoes through a food processor using the shred disk. Wring out any moisture from the potato shreds using cheesecloth, tea towel, and or nut milk bag.
2. In a large bowl, toss the potato shreds with bacon, scallions, salt, and pepper.

3. Heat a large pan over medium heat until very hot, about 5 minutes.

4. Add about 1/2 cup of shredded potato mixture to the pan, and then flatten using a spatula. Drizzle a portion of the melted butter on it. Cook until the bottom of the hash brown patty is crispy, about 5 minutes. Flip the patty and cook until the bottom side is crispy, about 5 minutes. Drain on a paper towel. Work in batches and repeat for the remainder of the hash brown mixture.

11. Curried Omelette

Prep Time: 10 Minutes

Cook Time: 15 Minutes

Servings: 1

Ingredients

- 3 eggs beaten
- 3 cups broccoli florets (about 5 ounces)
- 1 ounce sun-dried tomatoes chopped
- 2 tablespoons olive oil
- 2 tablespoons water
- 2 teaspoons curry powder
- 1/4 teaspoon salt
- 1/4 teaspoon pepper

Instructions

1. Heat olive oil on an 8-inch pan over medium heat. Add broccoli, curry powder, and water. Mix well. Cook until the broccoli is really tender, about 10 minutes, stirring frequently. Transfer broccoli to a plate.

2. Add more olive oil to the pan if it's dry. Combine beaten eggs with salt and pepper, and pour over the pan. Immediately add sun-dried tomatoes over the liquid eggs, evenly distributing them. Lift up the edges of the eggs to allow liquid eggs to run underneath. Cook until the bottom layer of eggs is solid, then flip the omelette.

3. Add broccoli back to the pan over the omelette. Fold the omelette over the broccoli. Optionally, you can add shredded cheese or garnish with parsley. Serve immediately.

Prep Time: 00 Minutes

Cook Time: 30 Minutes

Servings: 3

Ingredients

- Olive oil 2 TBS
- Chicken breasts or thighs cut in small bite sized pieces 400 g/14 oz
- 1 small onion 70 g
- Red and green or yellow bell peppers 220 g/7.7 oz
- Mushrooms cut in smaller pieces 150 g/5.3 oz
- 1 large zucchini 330 g/11.6 oz
- Crushed tomato or tomato sauce ¼ cup/50 ml
- Water or vegetable broth ¼ cup/50 ml
- Salt to taste
- Freshly ground pepper to taste
- Dried basil 1 tsp
- Dried oregano 1 tsp
- Turmeric powder 1 tsp
- Red paprika 1 tsp

TOPPING

- Feta cheese 100 g/3.5 oz
- Lemon juice 1 small lemon
- Extra virgin olive oil to drizzle

Instructions

1. In a large pan or a large skillet heat 2 TBS olive oil.
2. Cook chicken meat on a hot oil until golden brown on the edges and cooked. When cooked remove it from the skillet and set it aside on a plate.
3. On a remaining fat saute onion until translucent and golden brown.
4. When onion translucent, add mushrooms, peppers and zucchini. Add salt, pepper and spices and stir until veggies stat to get golden brown color on the edges and coated in spices.
5. Put back cooked chicken meat and add crushed tomato and ¼ cup water and stir.
6. When vegetables cooked to your liking remove from the heat and serve.
7. On top you can put feta cheese or goat cheese and drizzle with extra virgin olive oil and lemon juice.
8. Enjoy!

Prep Time: 00 Minutes

Cook Time: 45 Minutes

Servings: 5

Ingredients

- Lard or avocado oil for frying ⅔ cup/120 g/4.3 oz
- Chicken breast cut into schnitzels 500 g/17.7 oz
- 3 eggs beaten

Keto Meat Seasoning Mixture

- Salt 2 tsp
- Freshly ground pepper ¼ tsp
- Powdered garlic ½ tsp
- Ground paprika 1 tsp

Keto Schnitzel Coating Mixture

- Peanut flour defatted ½ cup/40 g/1.4 oz
- Almond flour or blanched almond meal ¼ cup/25 g/0.9 oz
- Grated parmesan cheese or Grana Padano 1 cup/100 g/3.5 oz

Optional For Serving

- Slices of lemon, chopped parsley or spring onion

Instructions

1. Prepare seasoning mixture. In a small bowl or in a small jar combine all the spices for seasoning.
2. Prepare whisked eggs in one bowl. Add a pinch of salt in eggs mixture.
3. Prepare coating/breading mixture in second plate.
4. Season the meat. Sprinkle each schnitzel from both sides with seasoning mixture to taste.
5. Each schnitzel dip into coating/breading mixture, coating both sides.
6. Next dip into the egg mixture coating both sides.
7. Then dip again into coating mixture to coat both sides with coating mixture.
8. Heat the lard or other healthy frying fat/oil and when start boiling on a medium high temperature (165 C/330 F) fry schnitzel for 2 - 3 minutes on each side until they become deep golden brown. Transfer to a plate lined with a paper towel.
9. Serve immediately with salad, slices of fresh lemon, cauliflower mash or with creamed spinach.

Prep Time: 10 Minutes

Cook Time: 20 Minutes

Servings: 4

Ingredients

- 1 zucchini, sliced to thin rounds 330g/11.64 oz
- Medium onion, thinly sliced 60 g/2.11 oz
- Large egg
- Salt and pepper to taste
- Paprika 1 tsp
- Almond flour ⅔ cup/70 g/2.46 oz
- Coconut flour 1 TBS/15 g/0.53 oz
- Mineral water 50 ml/3.5 TBS
- Spices to sprinkle on top:
- Paprika: 1 tsp
- Curry 1 tsp
- Parmesan cheese ¼ cup/25 g/0.88 oz
- Olive oil to sprinkle on top when baked (optional)

Instructions

1. Preheat the oven to 375°F (190°C).

2. Slice zucchini to thin rounds and thinly slice the onion.

3. In a mixing bowl, combine sliced zucchini and onion with a 2 pinches of salt, pinch of pepper & 1 teaspoon paprika. Toss them together until evenly distributed.

4. in a separate bowl whisk the egg, salt, almond flour, coconut flour & mineral water.

5. Mix everything thoroughly until a well-combined mixture is formed.

6. Combine with prepared zucchini and onion and distribute on a sheet pan layered with a parchment paper.

7. Sprinkle the top with 1 teaspoon of curry, 1 teaspoon of paprika, and grated ¼ cup of parmesan cheese. It will give your zucchinella delightful taste and a golden, crispy crust.

8. Place the baking dish in the preheated oven and bake for approximately 20 minutes or until the top turns golden brown and the zucchinella is cooked.

9. Remove the zucchinella from the oven and allow it to cool slightly. Cut it into desired portions and serve it as a side dish or as a main course alongside a fresh salad. This low-carb delight is perfect for lunch, dinner, or

even as a snack with a sour cream or similar dipping sauce.

Prep Time: 10 Minutes

Cook Time: 10 Minutes

Servings: 4

Ingredients

- Chicken thigh fillets, skinless & boneless 520 g/18.34 oz

FOR MARINADE

- Olive oil 1.5 TBS
- Lemon juice 2 TBS
- Powdered garlic ½ tsp
- Cumin ½ tsp
- Paprika 1 tsp
- Coriander 1 tsp
- Cardamon1 tsp
- Black pepper to taste
- Salt 1.5 teaspoon or more to taste
- SAUCE (optional)
- Sour cream 1 cup
- Powdered garlic ¼ tsp

- Cumin ½ tsp
- Lemon juice 1 TBS
- Pepper to taste
- Salt to taste

FOR SPICY OPTION

- Crushed chili pepper or cayenne to taste

FOR COOKING

- Olive oil 3 TBS

Instructions

1. Put the chicken thigh fillets in a large bowl.
2. In a small bowl mix together dry spices, pepper and salt and sprinkle on top of the meat.
3. Add olive oil and lemon juice, and stir everything to coat the meat well. Cover and marinate in the refrigerator for at least 30 minutes (or up to overnight). For the fast version, just skip this step of waiting.
4. Preheat your grill pan or skillet to medium-high heat and add olive oil.

5. Cook the first side of the meat for 4 to 8 minutes. Turn and cook the other side for 4 to 5 minutes (second side takes less time to cook).

6. Remove chicken from the grill pan or the skillet and cover with foul. Set aside to rest for 5 minutes.

7. Slice the chicken and seve with your favorite salads, keto tortilla, keto flatbread or cauliflower rice and add on top few tablespoons of the white sauce.

8. Serve and enjoy!

Prep Time: 10 Minutes

Cook Time: 30 Minutes

Servings: 4

Ingredients

VEGETABLE PIE FILLING

- Olive oil 1 or 2 TBS
- 1 medium onion 110 g/4 oz
- 1 small eggplant 160 g/5.6 oz
- Red bell pepper 100 g/3.5 oz
- 1 medium zucchini 190 g/6.7 oz
- Minced garlic clove
- Black olives 8 pieces/35 g/1.23 oz
- Crushed tomato ½ cup/100 g/3.5 oz
- 1 egg
- Salt ½ - 1 tsp
- Freshly ground pepper to taste
- Dried oregano 1 tsp
- Dried basil 1 tsp
- Balsamic vinegar 1 tsp

KETO SAVORY PIE CRUST

- Shredded mozzarella 2 cups/200 g/7 oz
- Almond flour 1 cup/100 g/3.5 oz
- Cream cheese 1 TBS
- Baking powder ½ tp
- Pinch salt
- Dried oregano 1 tsp
- Dried basil ½ tsp
- Pinch powdered garlic
- Powdered paprika ¼ tsp
- Crushed chili pinch (optional)

OPTIONAL TOPPING

- Fresh arugula 1 cup
- Fresh goat cheese or feta cheese 100 g/3.5 oz

Instructions

PREPARE VEGETABLE PIE FILLING

1. Heat 1 or 2 TBS of olive oil on a pan.
2. Add chopped onion on a hot oil and cook until golden brown and caramelized.

3. When onion is caramelized add eggplant cut in a small pieces, stir for 2 - 3 minutes.

4. Add red bell pepper chopped, stir for 2-3 minutes.

5. At the end add zucchini cut in small cubes, black olives cut into small pieces.

6. Season with salt, pepper, minced garlic clove and herbs.

7. Stir everything, add crushed tomatoes, 1 TBS of balsamic vinegar and 1 egg.

8. Remove from the heat and set aside until you prepare keto pie crust dough.

SAVORY KETO PIE CRUST

1. In a microwave safe bowl combine shredded mozzarella with a pinch of salt, 1 TBS of cream cheese, baking powder, almond flour and Mediterranean herbs like oregano and basil.

2. Optionally you can add a pinch of garlic and chili flakes or powdered paprika.

3. Stir everything and microwave for 45 seconds, take it out from the microwave, stir until all well combined.

4. Microwave for another 30 seconds.

5. After microwaving stir with the spoon until all the ingredients are combined, knead until keto dough is formed.

6. If it's not possible to knead, microwave for 30 to 45 seconds more.

7. Press the dough into the greased 25 cm/10 inch diameter pie dish and form the pie shell

ASSEMBLING KETO MEDITERRANEAN PIE

1. Turn on the oven to 180 C/350 F.
2. Put the vegetable filling into the keto pie dough shell.
3. Bake the pie in a preheated oven on 180 C for 15 - 20 minutes or until its golden brown on the edges.
4. Serve warm with arugula and goat cheese or feta cheese.
5. Enjoy!

Prep Time: 00 Minutes

Cook Time: 30 Minutes

Servings: 12

Ingredients

KETO ALMOND CRUST

- Ground almonds or almond meal 1.5 cup/160 g/5.64 oz
- Coconut flour 3 TBS/24 g/0.85 oz
- Erythritol or other low carb sweetener ¼ cup
- Softened butter 100 g/3.7 oz
- Pinch of salt
- Cinnamon ½ tsp

KETO CREAM FILLING

- Mascarpone cheese 1 cup/250 g/8.8 oz
- Heavy whipping cream ½ cup/100 ml
- 2 eggs
- Low carb sweetener (erythritol) 6 - 8 TBS
- Vanilla extract 1 tsp
- Cinnamon 1 tsp

CHERRIES

- Unsweetened cherries fresh or defrosted ⅔ cup/120 g/4.23 oz

DECORATION

- Melted sugar free white chocolate 10 g/0.35 oz
- Heavy whipping cream ½ cup/100 ml + powdered erythritol 2 TBS

Instructions

KETO ALMOND CRUST

1. Preheat the oven to 180 C/350 F.
2. Combine all ingredients together in a food processor or with your hands to get the dough.
3. Press in the dough into the greased 25 cm/10 inch diameter pie dish.
4. Bake in a preheated oven on 180 C/350 F for 10 to 15 minutes or until golden brown on the edges.
5. Leave it to rest for 15 minutes before you pour the filling.
6. If crust is puffed, press it gently with a spoon to make it flat.

KETO CREAM FILLING

1. Just mix all ingredients together until you get smooth filling. It will be liquid, don't worry, after baking and cooling in the fridge it will become firm.
2. When mixture is smooth, pour it on a baked pie crust.
3. Spread the cherries on top and bake in a preheated oven on 180 C/350 F for 30 minutes.
4. Leave it in the fridge for few hours to cool completely.

DECORATION (OPTIONAL)

1. Decorate the pie with some whipped heavy whipping cream and drizzle with melted sugar free white chocolate.
2. Decorate just before the serving.
3. Enjoy!

Prep Time: 00 Minutes

Cook Time: 20 Minutes

Servings: 4

Ingredients

CHICKEN WITH PEANUT BUTTER SAUCE

- Chicken breasts or chicken thighs cut in small cubes 450 g/16 oz
- Olive oil, lard or ghee 2 TBS

SPICES

- Salt to taste
- Pepper to taste
- Powdered garlic ¼ tsp
- Curry powder 1 tsp
- Cayenne pepper ¼ tsp
- Ground smoked paprika 1 tsp
- Turmeric ½ tsp
- Crushed chili pepper to taste
- Chicken or beef broth 1 cup

- Unsweetened peanut butter 2 TBS

- Heavy whipping cream ¼ cup/60 ml

FRIED CAULIFLOWER

- Olive oil 1 TBS

- 1 small onion 15 g

- Riced cauliflower 4 cups/450 g/16 oz

- Salt to taste

- Pepper to taste

- 1 egg

GARNISH (optional)

- Crushed peanuts

- Cilantro/coriander leaves

- Crushed chili

- Fresh cucumbers

- Slices of lemon or lime

Instructions

CHICKEN WITH PEANUT BUTTER SAUCE

1. Combine all the spices together in a bowl or a plate and coat chicken meat cut in small cubes in spice mix.

2. Heat the lard, olive oil or ghee and cook chicken meat coated in spices until meat is golden brown on the edges.

3. When meat golden brown, add broth, heavy whipping cream and peanut butter.

4. Stir everything and cook covered for 10 to 15 minutes on a medium heat.

FRIED CAULIFLOWER INSTRUCTIONS

1. Fry finely diced onion on hot olive oil.

2. When onion translucent and caramelized add rice cauliflower, salt and pepper to taste.

3. Stir cauliflower and fry until all the water is gone.

4. When cauliflower is fried, add one egg and stir until egg is completely fried and combined with cauliflower.

5. Serve hot as a side dish to chicken with peanut butter sauce.

6. Enjoy!

Prep Time: 10 Minutes

Cook Time: 20 Minutes

Servings: 5

Ingredients

- Olive oil or avocado oil 2 TBS
- Chicken meat (chicken breasts or chicken tights) cut into small cubes 600g/21 oz
- 3 L eggs
- Green peas ⅔ cup/100g/3.5 oz
- 1 small carrot cut in cubes 50g/1.8 oz
- 1 celery stalk cut in small pieces (optional) 20 g/0.7 oz
- 1 spring onion cut in small pieces 20 g/0.7 oz
- Riced cauliflower drained 2.5 cup/360 g/12.5 oz
- Salt 1 teaspoon or to taste
- Soy sauce or coconut aminos 2 TBS
- Powdered garlic 1 pinch
- Turmeric ½ tsp
- Sesame oil to taste
- Garnish (optional)
- Cilantro leaves

- Spring onion

Instructions

1. Prepare all ingredients before you start frying. Cut all vegetables and meat to small cubes.
2. Heat olive oil or avocado oil on a high heat in a skillet or a large pan.
3. Cook chicken for 5 minutes or until completely cooked stirring occasionally. Chicken should be golden brown on the edges. When cooked, transfer chicken meat to a plate.
4. Reduce the heat and pour beaten eggs on a pan and scramble for a minute. Cut scrambled eggs to a smaller pieces and transfer on a plate with meat.
5. If needed, clean the skillet with a paper towel and add more olive oil.
6. Boost the heat to high and cook chopped carrot, spring onion and optional celery, stir and when start to be brown add well drained cauliflower rice and peas.
7. Cook veggies with rice until start to be brown. Don't overcook it, it should be al dente, firm to bite and shouldn't lose the form.

8. When vegetables with cauliflower rice is cooked add salt, pepper, soy sauce or coconut aminos and other spices and herbs, stir well and add cooked chicken and scrambled eggs.

9. When finished drizzle with sesame oil and garnish with fresh cilantro leaves or chopped spring onion.

10. Enjoy!

Prep Time: 00 Minutes

Cook Time: 30 Minutes

Servings: 6

Ingredients

EGGPLANT

- Eggplant 400 g/14 oz
- Salt 1 tsp

MOUSSAKA MEAT SAUCE

- Olive oil 1 TBS
- Ground beef 450 g/16 oz
- Onion 50 g/1.7 oz
- Sugar free tomato sauce ½ cup
- Tomato paste 1 TBS
- Water or beef broth ½ cup
- Salt to taste
- Pepper to taste
- Powdered garlic ¼ tsp
- Cinnamon ¼ tsp
- Oregano ½ tsp

- Basil ½ tsp
- 1 bay leaf

KETO BECHAMEL SAUCE

- Cream cheese or mascarpone cheese 200 g/7 oz
- 1 M egg
- Pinch of salt
- Pepper to taste
- Pinch of nutmeg
- Pinch of powdered garlic

TOPPING

- Parmesan cheese 2 TBS

Instructions

PREPARE EGGPLANT

1. Slice eggplant to thin slices.
2. Salt it generously and leave it for 10 minutes to sweat in the bowl.
3. After 10 minutes rinse it well with a plenty of water.
4. Dry eggplant and put it on a sheet pan on a piece of parchment paper.

5. Bake for 10 to 20 minutes in a preheated oven with vent on 180 C/360 F or until slightly softened and browned.

MEAT SAUCE PREPARATION

1. Heat 1 TBS of olive oil.
2. Sauté chopped onion on hot olive oil until translucent.
3. Add ground meat and stir until browned.
4. Add salt, pepper, powdered garlic, herbs and stir.
5. Pour tomato sauce, tomato paste and water or broth and stir.
6. Put the bay leaf and leave it to cook uncovered until water dissolved. Stir occasionally.
7. While cooking the sauce, preheat the oven to 180 C/360 F.

PREPARE KETO BECHAMEL SAUCE

1. Mix cream cheese or mascarpone cheese with 1 M egg. Add pinch of salt, pepper, powdered garlic and a pinch of nutmeg. Whisk or mix until nicely combined.

ASSEMBLING MOUSSAKA

2. Place half of the eggplant slices on the bottom of deep lasagna dish and top with meat sauce.
3. Place another half of eggplant slices on the sauce layer.
4. Pour everything with keto bechamel sauce.

TOPPING

1. Sprinkle with 2 TBS of parmesan cheese.
2. Bake in preheated oven with vent on 180 C/360 F for 15 - 30 minutes (depends on your oven) or until golden brown crust is formed on top.
3. Serve keto moussaka hot with some leafy green salad.
4. Enjoy!

Prep Time: 00 Minutes

Cook Time: 30 Minutes

Servings: 6

Ingredients

- Ingredients for fried keto chicken strips
- Chicken tenders 600 g
- Lard or coconut oil 1 cup for frying
- Ingredients for keto batter
- 2 L eggs
- Coconut flour 5 TBS/35 g/1.24 oz
- Sesame flour 5 TBS/25 g/0.88 oz
- Liquid yogurt ⅓ cup/100 ml
- Heavy whipping cream ⅓ cup/100 ml
- Salt ½ tsp
- Optional spices and additions to your taste
- Ground pepper
- Red paprika
- Powdered garlic
- Chili pepper

- Dried or fresh chopped herbs (parsley, basil, oregano...)
- Parmesan cheese shredded
- Sesame seeds

Instructions

1. How to make keto chicken fingers?
2. Prepare chicken strips/ chicken tenders and season with salt and pepper to your taste. You can add other other optional spices.
3. Prepare keto batter.
4. How to make keto batter?
5. Whisk the eggs and set aside.
6. Mix all dry ingredients - coconut flour and sesame flour with salt, spices and herbs you like.
7. Add dry mixture to eggs, add yogurt and heavy whipping cream and whisk until you get smooth keto batter.
8. Frying procedure
9. Dip each chicken tender into prepared keto batter and put it on a hot lard or coconut oil.
10. Fry it on a medium heat until golden brown and meat completely cooked. Be careful and don't fry it on a very

high heat and too hot lard or oil because it might burn
and become dry.

21. Creamy Keto Chicken Casserole

Prep Time: 15 Minutes

Cook Time: 30 Minutes

Servings: 6

Ingredients

- Chicken breast, tenders, or chicken thighs (without skin) 770 g/27 oz
- Salt to taste
- Ground paprika 1 tsp
- Pepper to taste
- Onion 80 g/2.8 oz
- Garlic ¼ tsp
- Mushrooms cut in halves 500 g/17.6 oz
- Heavy whipping cream 1 cup/220 ml
- Parmesan cheese ½ cup/50 g/0.16 oz (¼ cup for chicken and ¼ cup for the sauce)
- Chicken broth or water 1 cup/220 ml
- Lemon juice 2 TBS
- Nutmeg ¼ tsp
- Parsley chopped 1 TBS

Instructions

1. Season the chicken with salt, pepper, ground paprika, and sprinkle both sides with grated parmesan cheese.
2. Sautee chicken in a skillet or pan in hot olive oil, until golden brown.
3. Transfer the chicken to the casserole baking dish 26 x 17 x 7 cm/10 x 7 x 3 inch.
4. In the remaining oil sautee chopped onion and garlic.
5. When the onion is golden brown and caramelized, add chopped mushrooms and a pinch of salt and saute until soft and golden brown on the edges.
6. Add heavy whipping cream, chicken broth or water, lemon juice, nutmeg, and parmesan cheese. Stir it well and cook for 2 to 3 minutes.
7. Add it to the casserole and combine it with chicken.
8. Bake covered in a preheated oven on 175C/350 for 30 minutes.
9. When baked, garnish with parsley and serve with salad and mashed cauliflower.
10. Enjoy!

Prep Time: 10 Minutes

Cook Time: 45 Minutes

Servings: 5

Ingredients

- Lard 2 TBS
- Onion chopped 70 g/2.50 oz
- Savoy cabbage chopped 550 g/19 oz
- Beef cubes 450 g/16 oz
- Kohlrabi cut to cubes 100 g/3.50 oz (optional)
- Carrot cut to small cubed 20 g/0.70 oz
- Tomato sauce ¼ cup/50 g/1.80 oz
- Turmeric ½ TBS
- Salt 1 teaspoon or more to taste
- Freshly ground pepper to taste
- Ground paprika 1 TBS
- Basil pinch
- Water or beef broth 2.5 cups

Instructions

1. Melt lard or heat olive oil.

2. Sauté chopped onion until translucent and golden brown.

3. Add beef meat cubes and stir until browned on the edges. This is very important step because it gives flavor.

4. When meat browned add savoy cabbage chopped into small pieces and stir for few minutes until starts to wilt.

5. Add tomato, carrot and turnip cut in small cubes, spices, and salt and water or broth.

6. Stir and cook covered for 1.5 h on low to medium heat or in the instant pot for at least 30 - 45 minutes. Longer you cook its better!

7. Serve and enjoy!

Prep Time: 10 Minutes

Cook Time: 25 Minutes

Servings: 4

Ingredients

- Olive oil 2 TBS
- 1 small onion 77g/2.7oz
- Garlic 2 - 3 cloves
- Red pepper finely chopped 120 g/4.23 oz
- Jalapeno green or yellow finely 110 g/3.88 oz
- Chopped tomatoes in tomato juice canned or fresh 1 can/400 g/14.11 oz
- Chicken broth or water 4 cups/600 ml
- Chicken breast 490 g/17.28 oz
- Oregano 1 TBS
- Paprika 1 TBS
- Powdered garlic ½ TBS
- Cumin ½ TBS
- Salt 1 tsp
- Pepper ½ tsp

TOPPINGS

- Keto tortilla chips
- Avocado
- Lime slices
- Cilantro
- Sour cream
- Shredded cheese (Monterey Jack)

Instructions

1. Heat thc olive oil.
2. Saute finely chopped onion until translucent, golden brown and caramelized.
3. Add finely chopped red pepper and jalapeno, stir for 30 sec, and add garlic.
4. Make some space for chicken, add whole chicken meat and brown it on each side for 20 seconds.
5. Add broth or water, chopped tomatoes, salt and spices.
6. Stir and set it to pressure cooking for 25 minutes.
7. If cooking on the stove, cook 45 min., and in the slow cooker 6 to 8 hours.
8. When cooked in the instant pot, release the pressure, take the chicken out to shred it. After shredding, put it back in the pot, stir and serve.

9. Add some toppings - definitelly keto tortilla chips, avocado, slices of lime, and if you like you can add sour cream, shredded cheese and cilantro.

Prep Time: 10 Minutes

Cook Time: 10 Minutes

Servings: 4

Ingredients

- Cauliflower florets 360 g/12.7 oz
- Salt to taste
- Pepper to taste
- Turmeric ½ tsp
- Powdered garlic ¼ tsp
- Grated parmesan or Grana Padano ¼ cup/25 g
- Shredded mozzarella 1 cup/110 g

Instructions

1. Preheat the oven to 190°C/375°F.
2. Prepare a baking sheet with parchment paper.
3. Cut the head of cauliflower into florets and put them into boiling water with a pinch of salt for 3 to 5 minutes.
4. After 5 minutes place them on a prepared baking sheet. Crush them with the bottom of the glass.

5. Season with salt, pepper, and spices, and cover with cheese. Make sure to coat everything.

6. Bake in a preheated oven for 10-15 minutes, or until the cauliflower is roasted, cheese melted, and golden-brown on top.

7. Once the cheesy cauliflower is roasted, remove it from the oven.

8. Serve with your favorite sauce, and meat as a keto side dish, or as a keto vegetarian cauliflower dinner with cheese sauce.

Prep Time: 00 Minutes

Cook Time: 30 Minutes

Servings: 5

Ingredients

- Cod fish fillets fresh or frozen (you can use instead other white fish like snapper, monkfish or salmon) 450 g/16 oz
- Olive oil or coconut oil 2 TBS
- Onion finely chopped 70 g/2.5 oz
- Garlic 1 or 2 cloves
- Carrot 1 small 50 g/1.7 oz
- Green peas ¼ cup/25 g/0.8 oz
- Cauliflower 220 g/7.7 oz
- Zucchini 2 medium 300g/10.5 oz
- Full fat coconut milk 1 can/400 ml
- Fish or vegetable broth 2 cups/400 ml
- Salt to taste
- Pepper to taste
- Dried basil 1 tsp
- Turmeric 1 tsp

- Nutmeg powder ¼ tsp

TO SERVE

- Fresh cilantro or parsley
- Lime juice to taste

Instructions

1. In a large pot on a high heat, melt the oil and fry finely chopped onion.
2. When onion is translucent and golden brown, add minced garlic, carrot cut in small cubes and cauliflower cut in small pieces.
3. Stir and cook the vegetables until it start to be golden brown on the edges.
4. Add coconut milk and broth, salt, pepper, basil, turmeric and nutmeg, stir.
5. Bring it to simmer and cook for 10 minutes.
6. After 10 minutes add fish cut in small pieces, peas and zucchini cut in small pieces.
7. Cook for 10 minutes.
8. Serve with fresh cilantro or parsley leaves, crushed chili and fresh lime juice.
9. Enjoy!

Prep Time: 00 Minutes

Cook Time: 20 Minutes

Servings: 4

Ingredients

- Coconut oil 2 TBS
- White fish fillets (cod, hake, John Dory, tilapia or snapper) 450 g/16 oz
- Salt to taste
- Freshly ground pepper to taste
- Garlic clove
- Full fat canned coconut milk 1 cup/200 ml
- Powdered turmeric ½ tsp
- Dried basil 1 tsp
- Lime juice of 1 lime

OPTIONAL

- Crushed chili
- Fresh cilantro leaves

Instructions

1. In a large pan or a skillet, heat the coconut oil and minced garlic clove.
2. Season the fish fillets from both sides with a pinch of salt and freshly ground pepper to taste.
3. When the oil is hot cook fish fillets from both sides. First cook on a fish flesh side and when cooked, turn fillets to skin side and cook until completely cooked. While fish is cooking add juice of ½ lime.
4. In a small bowl whisk full fat coconut milk with 1 teaspoon of turmeric, pinch of salt and pepper to taste and pour over the cooked fish fillets.
5. Sprinkle with dried basil and add another half of lime juice.
6. Cook everything and bring it so simmer.
7. When starts to simmer cook for 5 minutes and serve warm.
8. Serve with fried cauliflower rice.
9. Optionally garnish with fresh cilantro and crushed chili.
10. Enjoy!

Prep Time: 10 Minutes

Cook Time: 20 Minutes

Servings: 6

Ingredients

- Coconut oil 2 TBS
- Fish fillets (cod, snapper, halibut, hake, salmon or John Dory) 475 g/16.7 oz
- Shrimp 200 g/7 oz
- 1 small onion finely diced 70 g/2.5 oz
- 1 red pepper/capsicum 100 g/3.5 oz
- 2 cloves garlic minced
- Full fat canned coconut milk 1 can/400 ml/14 oz
- Crushed tomatoes 1 cup/200 ml/7 oz
- Fish broth/stock or water 1 cup/200 ml/7 oz
- Salt to taste
- Freshly ground pepper to taste
- Cumin powder 1 tsp
- Ground red paprika 1 TBS
- Curry powder 1 TBS
- Cayenne pepper 1 tsp

- Lime juice 2 TBS

GARNISH

- Cilantro leaved
- Crushed chili
- Lime juice

Instructions

1. Season fish cut in small bite sized pieces and shrimp with freshly ground pepper and salt in a bowl.
2. Heat 2 TBS of coconut oil in a large skillet over high heat. Add fish and shrimp and cook until cooked and just a little golden brown on the edges. When cooked, remove fish and shrimp from the skillet and set aside on a plate.
3. Reduce the heat to medium high and on a remaining oil add onion and cook until onion translucent and golden brown, add capsicum cut in small slices and minced garlic and cook until capsicum start to get grown color on the edges. It will take 1 or 2 minutes.
4. Add crushed tomato, coconut milk and broth or water. Stir well, add spices, salt and pepper, stir and bring it to simmer. Cook for 10 - 15 minutes.

5. After 10 to 15 minutes return fish and shrimp and cook for 2 to 3 minutes.

6. Add lime juice, stir and serve.

7. Garnish with crushed chili and cilantro leaves.

8. Enjoy!

Prep Time: 10 Minutes

Cook Time: 20 Minutes

Servings: 5

Ingredients

- Lard or olive oil 1 TBS
- Finely sliced bacon 50 g/1.77 oz
- Onion 70 g/2.47 oz
- Ground beef 450 g/1 lb
- Mushrooms 200 g/7 oz
- Red pepper chopped 1 cup/150 g/5.3 oz
- Cottage cheese 2 TBS/20 g/0.7 oz
- Feta cheese 3 TBS/30 g/1 oz
- 2 large eggs
- Powdered garlic ½ tsp
- Ground smoked paprika 1 tsp
- Salt 1.5 tsp
- Freshly ground pepper to taste
- Dried basil 1 tsp
- Chilli pepper to taste
- Freshly chopped parsley

Instructions

1. Fry bacon on a hot lard and when start to be translucent add finely chopped onion.
2. When onion is translucent, add ground beef and stir occasionally until golden brown.
3. When beef is golden brown add mushrooms and finely chopped red peppers or capsicum and stir.
4. Season with salt, pepper, ground red paprika, dried basil, powdered garlic and chili to taste, stir and cook until mushrooms are wilted.
5. Add cottage cheese and feta cheese, stir well and cook for few minutes with occasional stirring until the majority of water from veggies and cheese is gone.
6. Put on top 2 or more eggs and cook it covered until eggs are cooked to your taste.
7. Garnish with finely diced parsley.
8. Serve hot and enjoy.

Prep Time: 00 Minutes

Cook Time: 20 Minutes

Servings: 4

Ingredients

CHICKEN WITH PEANUT BUTTER SAUCE

- Chicken breasts or chicken thighs cut in small cubes 450 g/16 oz
- Olive oil, lard or ghee 2 TBS

SPICES

- Salt to taste
- Pepper to taste
- Powdered garlic ¼ tsp
- Curry powder 1 tsp
- Cayenne pepper ¼ tsp
- Ground smoked paprika 1 tsp
- Turmeric ½ tsp
- Crushed chili pepper to taste
- Chicken or beef broth 1 cup

- Unsweetened peanut butter 2 TBS
- Heavy whipping cream ¼ cup/60 ml

FRIED CAULIFLOWER

- Olive oil 1 TBS
- 1 small onion 15 g
- Riced cauliflower 4 cups/450 g/16 oz
- Salt to taste
- Pepper to taste
- 1 egg

GARNISH (optional)

- Crushed peanuts
- Cilantro/coriander leaves
- Crushed chili
- Fresh cucumbers
- Slices of lemon or lime

Instructions

CHICKEN WITH PEANUT BUTTER SAUCE

1. Combine all the spices together in a bowl or a plate and coat chicken meat cut in small cubes in spice mix.

2. Heat the lard, olive oil or ghee and cook chicken meat coated in spices until meat is golden brown on the edges.

3. When meat golden brown, add broth, heavy whipping cream and peanut butter.

4. Stir everything and cook covered for 10 to 15 minutes on a medium heat.

FRIED CAULIFLOWER INSTRUCTIONS

1. Fry finely diced onion on hot olive oil.

2. When onion translucent and caramelized add rice cauliflower, salt and pepper to taste.

3. Stir cauliflower and fry until all the water is gone.

4. When cauliflower is fried, add one egg and stir until egg is completely fried and combined with cauliflower.

5. Serve hot as a side dish to chicken with peanut butter sauce.

6. Enjoy!

Prep Time: 10 Minutes

Cook Time: 20 Minutes

Servings: 4

Ingredients

INGREDIENTS FOR THAI PORK TENDERLOIN

- Coconut oil or avocado oil 2 TBS
- Pork tenderloin 600 g/21 oz
- Baby spinach 100 g/3.5 oz
- 2 spring onions
- Oyster sauce 2 TBS
- Coconut aminos or soy sauce 2 TBS
- Salt to taste
- Pepper to taste
- Pinch of powdered garlic or 1 small clove crushed
- Pinch of powdered ginger or grated fresh ginger
- Pinch of dried chili
- Optional ingredients
- Toasted sesame seeds 1 TBS
- Toasted peanuts 1 TBS

- Sesame oil 1 TBS

INGREDIENTS FOR CAULIFLOWER RICE

- Riced cauliflower 400 g/14 oz
- 1 large egg
- Pinch of salt
- Pinch of pepper
- Optional ingredients
- Sesame oil 1 TBS
- Coconut aminos or soy sauce 1 TBS

Instructions

THAI PORK TENDERLOIN PROCEDURE

1. Heat oil in wok, pan or skillet over high heat.
2. Add pork meat cut in small cubes and cook for 5 - 8 minutes or until golden brown and cooked.
3. Add coconut aminos or soy sauce and oyster sauce, salt (be careful with salt because oyster sauce and aminos are salty), pepper, chili, garlic and ginger and stir well.
4. Add spring onion cut into 3 - 4 longer parts and baby spinach and stir until spinach wilted.
5. Serve immediately with fried cauliflower rice.

6. Drizzle with sesame oil and sprinkle with crushed toasted peanuts and toasted sesame seeds.

FRIED CAULIFLOWER RICE PROCEDURE

1. Heat the pan and add drained riced cauliflower on a hot pan.
2. Stir until the water from cauliflower is gone.
3. Stir 1 large egg into the cauliflower until combined and fried with cauliflower.
4. Add pinch of salt and pepper and optional 1 TBS of soy sauce or coconut aminos and sesame oil.
5. Enjoy!

www.ingramcontent.com/pod-product-compliance
Lightning Source LLC
Chambersburg PA
CBHW061005260726
48661CB00005B/2062